Keto Air Fryer Seafood Collection

Stay Healthy

with These Affordable Dishes

Lucy Grant

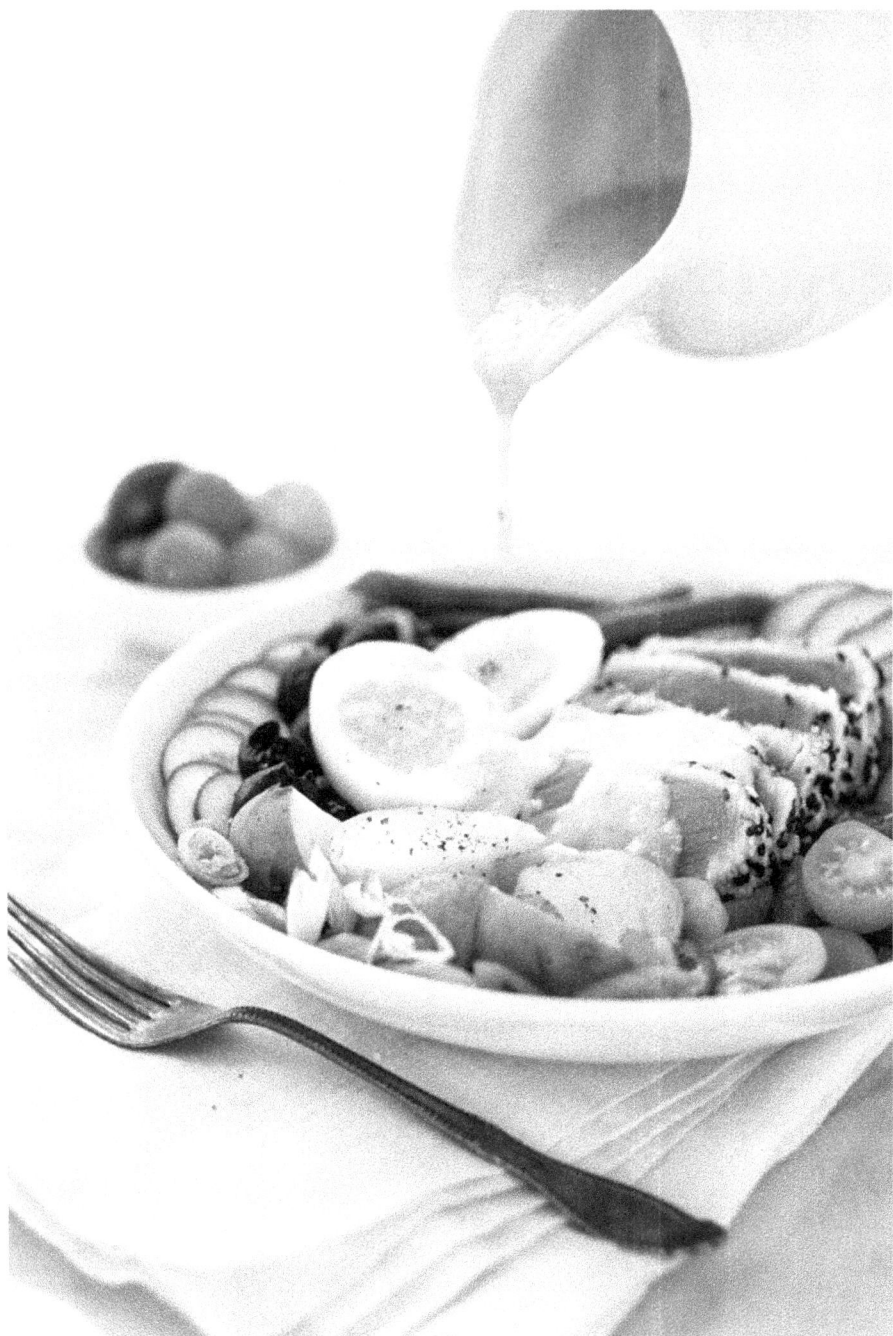

reader will render any resulting actions solely under their purview. There are no scenarios in which the publisher or the original author of this work can be in any fashion deemed liable for any hardship or damages that may befall them after undertaking information described herein.

Additionally, the information in the following pages is intended only for informational purposes and should thus be thought of as universal. As befitting its nature, it is presented without assurance regarding its prolonged validity or interim quality. Trademarks that are mentioned are done without written consent and can in no way be considered an endorsement from the trademark holder.

Table of Contents

Introduction

What's the difference between an air fryer and deep fryer? Air fryers bake food at a high temperature with a high-powered fan, while deep fryers cook food in a vat of oil that has been heated up to a specific temperature. Both cook food quickly, but an air fryer requires practically zero preheat time while a deep fryer can take upwards of 10 minutes. Air fryers also require little to no oil and deep fryers require a lot that absorb into the food. Food comes out crispy and juicy in both appliances, but don't taste the same, usually because deep fried foods are coated in batter that cook differently in an air fryer vs a deep fryer. Battered foods needs to be sprayed with oil before cooking in an air fryer to help them color and get crispy, while the hot oil soaks into the batter in a deep fryer. Flour-based batters and wet batters don't cook well in an air fryer, but they come out very well in a deep fryer.

The ketogenic diet is one such example. The diet calls for a very small number of carbs to be eaten. This means food such as rice, pasta, and other starchy vegetables like potatoes are off the menu. Even relaxed versions of the keto diet minimize carbs to a large extent and this compromises the goals of many dieters. They end up having to exert large amounts of willpower to follow the diet. This doesn't do them any favors since willpower is like a muscle. At some point, it tires and this is when the dieter goes right back to their old pattern of eating. I have personal experience with this. In terms of health benefits, the keto diet offers the most. The reduction of carbs forces your body to mobilize fat and this results in automatic fat loss and better health.

Feel free to mix and match the recipes you see in here and play around with them. Eating is supposed to be fun! Unfortunately, we've associated fun eating with unhealthy food. This doesn't have to be the case. The air fryer, combined with the Mediterranean diet, will make your mealtimes fun-filled again and full of taste. There's no grease and messy cleanups to deal with anymore. Are you excited yet?

You should be! You're about to embark on a journey full of air fried goodness!

Halibut Cakes with Horseradish Mayo

Prep + Cook Time: 20 minutes

4 Servings

INGREDIENTS

Halibut Cakes:

1 pound halibut

2 tablespoons olive oil

1/2 teaspoon cayenne pepper

1/4 teaspoon black pepper

Salt, to taste

2 tablespoons cilantro, chopped

1 shallot, chopped

2 garlic cloves, minced

1/2 cup Romano cheese, grated

1/2 cup breadcrumbs

1 egg, whisked

1 tablespoon Worcestershire sauce

Mayo Sauce:

1 teaspoon horseradish, grated

1/2 cup mayonnaise

DIRECTIONS

Start by preheating your Air Fryer to 380 degrees F.

Spritz the Air Fryer basket with cooking oil.

Mix all ingredients for the halibut cakes in a bowl; knead with your hands until everything is well incorporated.

Shape the mixture into equally sized patties.

Transfer your patties to the Air Fryer basket.

Cook the fish patties for 10 minutes, turning them over halfway through.

Mix the horseradish and mayonnaise.

Serve the halibut cakes with the horseradish mayo.

Sunday Fish with Sticky Sauce

Prep + Cook Time: 20 minutes

2 Servings

INGREDIENTS

1 pollack fillets

Salt and black pepper, to taste

1 tablespoon olive oil

1 cup chicken broth

2 tablespoons light soy sauce

1 tablespoon brown sugar

2 tablespoons butter, melted

1 teaspoon fresh ginger, minced

1 teaspoon fresh garlic, minced

2 corn tortillas

DIRECTIONS

Pat dry the pollack fillets and season them with salt and black pepper; drizzle the sesame oil all over the fish fillets.

Preheat the Air Fryer to 380 degrees F and cook your fish for 11 minutes.

Slice into bite-sized pieces.

Meanwhile, prepare the sauce.

Add the broth to a large saucepan and bring to a boil.

Add the soy sauce, sugar, butter, ginger, and garlic.

Reduce the heat to simmer and cook until it is reduced slightly.

Add the fish pieces to the warm sauce.

Serve on corn tortillas and enjoy!

Crusty Catfish with Sweet Potato Fries

Prep + Cook Time: 50 minutes

2 Servings

INGREDIENTS

1/2 pound catfish

1/2 cup bran cereal

1/4 cup parmesan cheese, grated

Sea salt and ground black pepper, to taste

1 teaspoon smoked paprika

1 teaspoon garlic powder

1/4 teaspoon ground bay leaf

1 egg

2 tablespoons butter, melted

4 sweet potatoes, cut French fries

DIRECTIONS

Pat the catfish dry with a kitchen towel.

Combine the bran cereal with the parmesan cheese and all spices in a shallow bowl.

Whisk the egg in another shallow bowl.

Dip the fish in the egg mixture and turn to coat evenly; then, dredge in the bran cereal mixture, turning a couple of times to coat evenly.

Spritz the Air Fryer basket with cooking spray.

Cook the catfish in the preheated Air Fryer at 390 degrees F for 10 minutes; turn them over and cook for 4 minutes more.

Then, drizzle the melted butter all over the sweet potatoes; cook them in the preheated Air Fryer at 380 degrees F for 30 minutes, shaking occasionally.

Serve over the warm fish fillets.

Enjoy!

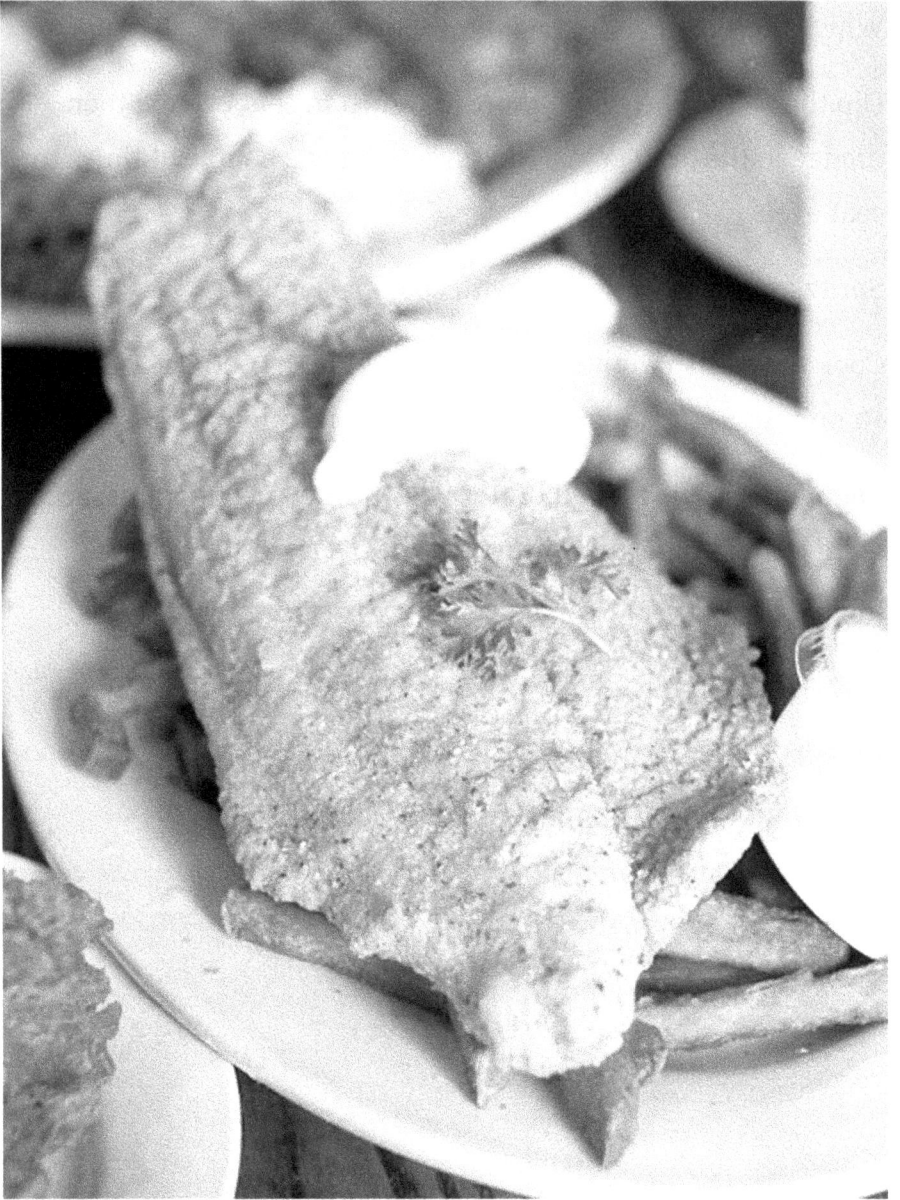

Easy Creamy Shrimp Nachos

Prep + Cook Time: 15 minutes

4 Servings

INGREDIENTS

1 pound shrimp, cleaned and deveined

1 tablespoon olive oil

2 tablespoons fresh lemon juice

1 teaspoon paprika

1/4 teaspoon cumin powder

1/2 teaspoon shallot powder

1/2 teaspoon garlic powder

Coarse sea salt and ground black pepper, to taste

1 9-ounce bag corn tortilla chips

1/4 cup pickled jalapeño, minced

1 cup Pepper Jack cheese, grated

1/2 cup sour cream

DIRECTIONS

Toss the shrimp with the olive oil, lemon juice, paprika, cumin powder, shallot powder, garlic powder, salt, and black pepper.

Cook in the preheated Air Fryer at 390 degrees F for 5 minutes.

Place the tortilla chips on the aluminum foil-lined cooking basket.

Top with the shrimp mixture, jalapeño and cheese.

Cook another 2 minutes or until cheese has melted.

Serve garnished with sour cream and enjoy!

Famous Tuna Niçoise Salad

Prep + Cook Time: 15 minutes

3 Servings

INGREDIENTS

1 pound tuna steak

Sea salt and ground black pepper, to taste

1/2 teaspoon red pepper flakes, crushed

1/4 teaspoon dried dill weed

1/2 teaspoon garlic paste

1 pound green beans, trimmed

2 handfuls baby spinach

2 handfuls iceberg lettuce, torn into pieces

1/2 red onion, sliced

1 cucumber, sliced

2 tablespoons lemon juice

1 tablespoon olive oil

1 teaspoon Dijon mustard

1 tablespoon balsamic vinegar 1 tablespoon roasted almonds, coarsely chopped

1 tablespoon fresh parsley, coarsely chopped

DIRECTIONS

Pat the tuna steak dry; toss your tuna with salt, black pepper, red pepper, dill and garlic paste.

Spritz your tuna with a nonstick cooking spray.

Cook the tuna steak at 400 degrees F for 5 minutes; turn your tuna steak over and continue to cook for 4 to 5 minutes more.

Then, add the green beans to the cooking basket.

Spritz green beans with a nonstick cooking spray.

Cook at 400 degrees F for 5 minutes, shaking the basket once or twice.

Cut your tuna into thin strips and transfer to a salad bowl; add in the green beans.

Then, add in the baby spinach, iceberg lettuce, onion and cucumber and toss to combine.

In a mixing bowl, whisk the lemon juice, olive oil, mustard and vinegar.

Dress the salad and garnish with roasted almonds and fresh parsley.

Serve and enjoy!

Classic Pancetta-Wrapped Scallops

Prep + Cook Time: 10 minutes

3 Servings

INGREDIENTS

1 pound sea scallops

1 tablespoon deli mustard

2 tablespoons soy sauce

1/4 teaspoon shallot powder

1/4 teaspoon garlic powder

1/2 teaspoon dried dill

Sea salt and ground black pepper, to taste

4 ounces pancetta slices

DIRECTIONS

Pat dry the sea scallops and transfer them to a mixing bowl.

Toss the sea scallops with the deli mustard, soy sauce, shallot powder, garlic powder, dill, salt and black pepper.

Wrap a slice of bacon around each scallop and transfer them to the Air Fryer cooking basket.

Cook in your Air Fryer at 400 degrees F for 4 minutes; turn them over and cook an additional 3 minutes.

Serve with hot sauce for dipping if desired.

Enjoy!

Fried Oysters with Kaffir Lime Sauce

Prep + Cook Time: 10 minutes

2 Servings

INGREDIENTS

8 fresh oysters, shucked

1/3 cup plain flour

1 egg

3/4 cup breadcrumbs

1/2 teaspoon Italian seasoning mix

1 lime, freshly squeezed

1 teaspoon coconut sugar

1 kaffir lime leaf, shredded

1 habanero pepper, minced

1 teaspoon olive oil

DIRECTIONS

Clean the oysters and set them aside.

Add the flour to a rimmed plate.

Whisk the egg in another rimmed plate.

Mix the breadcrumbs and Italian seasoning mix in a third plate.

Dip your oysters in the flour, shaking off the excess.

Then, dip them in the egg mixture and finally, coat your oysters with the breadcrumb mixture.

Spritz the breaded oysters with a nonstick cooking spray.

Cook your oysters in the preheated Air Fryer at 400 degrees F for 2 to 3 minutes, shaking the basket halfway through the cooking time.

Meanwhile, blend the remaining ingredients to make the sauce.

Serve the warm oysters with the kaffir lime sauce on the side.

Enjoy!

Spicy Curried King Prawns

Prep + Cook Time: 10 minutes

2 Servings

INGREDIENTS

12 king prawns, rinsed

1 tablespoon coconut oil

1/2 teaspoon piri piri powder

Salt and ground black pepper, to taste

1 teaspoon garlic paste

1 teaspoon onion powder

1/2 teaspoon cumin powder

1 teaspoon curry powder

DIRECTIONS

In a mixing bowl, toss all ingredient until the prawns are well coated on all sides.

Cook in the preheated Air Fryer at 360 degrees F for 4 minutes.

Shake the basket and cook for 4 minutes more.

Serve over hot rice if desired.

Enjoy!

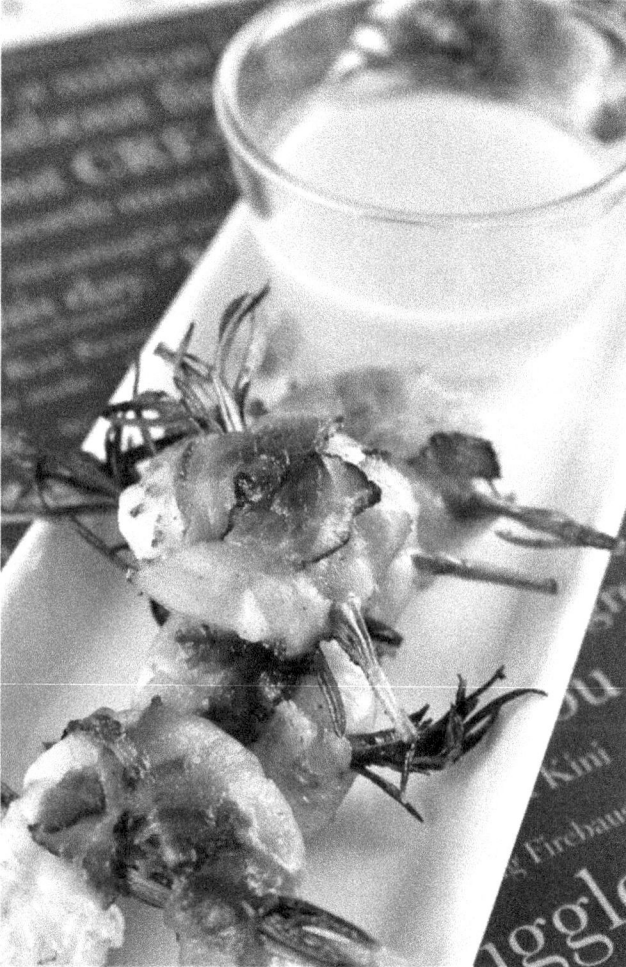

Grilled Salmon Steaks

Prep + Cook Time: 45 minutes

4 Servings

INGREDIENTS

2 cloves garlic, minced

4 tablespoons butter, melted

Sea salt and ground black pepper, to taste

1 teaspoon smoked paprika

1/2 teaspoon onion powder

1 tablespoon lime juice

1/4 cup dry white wine

4 salmon steaks

DIRECTIONS

Place all ingredients in a large ceramic dish.

Cover and let it marinate for 30 minutes in the refrigerator.

Arrange the salmon steaks on the grill pan.

Bake at 390 degrees for 5 minutes, or until the salmon steaks are easily flaked with a fork.

Flip the fish steaks, baste with the reserved marinade, and cook another 5 minutes.

Serve and enjoy!

Indian Famous Fish Curry

Prep + Cook Time: 25 minutes

4 Servings

INGREDIENTS

2 tablespoons sunflower oil

1/2 pound fish, chopped

2 red chilies, chopped

1 tablespoon coriander powder

1 teaspoon curry paste

1 cup coconut milk

Salt and white pepper, to taste

1/2 teaspoon fenugreek seeds

1 shallot, minced

1 garlic clove, minced

1 ripe tomato, pureed

DIRECTIONS

Preheat your Air Fryer to 380 degrees F; brush the cooking basket with 1 tablespoon of sunflower oil.

Cook your fish for 10 minutes on both sides.

Transfer to the baking pan that is previously greased with the remaining tablespoon of sunflower oil.

Add the remaining ingredients and reduce the heat to 350 degrees F.

Continue to cook an additional 10 to 12 minutes or until everything is heated through.

Enjoy!

Crispy Prawns in Bacon Wraps

Prep + Cook Time: 30 minutes

4 Servings

INGREDIENTS

8 bacon slices

8 jumbo prawns, peeled and deveined

DIRECTIONS

Wrap each prawn from head to tail with each bacon slice overlapping to keep the bacon in place.

Secure the ends with toothpicks.

Refrigerate for 15 minutes.

Preheat air fryer to 400 F.

Arrange the bacon-wrapped prawns on the greased frying basket and Bake for 8 minutes, turning once.

Serve hot.

Mango Shrimp Skewers with Hot Sauce

Prep + Cook Time: 20 minutes + marinating time

4 Servings

INGREDIENTS

20 small-sized shrimp, peeled and deveined

2 tbsp olive oil

½ tsp garlic powder

1 tsp mango powder

2 tbsp fresh lime juice Salt and black pepper to taste

2 tbsp fresh cilantro, chopped

1 garlic clove, minced

1 green onion, finely sliced

1 tbsp red chili flakes, crushed

4 tbsp olive oil

2 tbsp white wine vinegar

DIRECTIONS

In a bowl, mix garlic powder, mango powder, lime juice, salt, and black pepper.

Add the shrimp and toss to coat.

Cover and marinate for 20 minutes.

Soak wooden skewers in water for 15 minutes.

In a small dish, mix cilantro, minced garlic, green onion, chili flakes, olive oil, and champagne vinegar.

Preheat air fryer to 390 F.

Thread the marinated shrimp onto the skewers, drizzle with olive oil, and place in the frying basket.

AirFry for 5 minutes, shake the shrimp, and cook for 5 more minutes.

Serve the skewers with the cilantro sauce.

American Panko Fish Nuggets

Prep + Cook Time: 20 minutes

4 Servings

INGREDIENTS

1 lb fish fillets

1 lemon, juiced

Salt and black pepper to taste

1 tsp dried dill

4 tbsp mayonnaise

2 eggs, beaten

1 tbsp garlic powder

1 cup breadcrumbs

1 tsp paprika

DIRECTIONS

Preheat air fryer to 400 F.

Season the fish with salt and black pepper.

In a bowl, mix beaten eggs, lemon juice, and mayonnaise.

In a separate bowl, mix breadcrumbs, paprika, dill, and garlic powder.

Dredge the fillets in the egg mixture and then in the crumbs.

Place the fillets in the greased frying basket and AirFry for 15 minutes, flipping once halfway through.

Serve warm.

Golden Cod Fish Fillets

Prep + Cook Time: 20 minutes

4 Servings

INGREDIENTS

4 cod fillets

2 tbsp olive oil

2 eggs, beaten

1 cup breadcrumbs

A pinch of salt

1 cup flour

DIRECTIONS

Preheat air fryer to 390 F.

Mix breadcrumbs, olive oil, and salt in a bowl.

In another bowl, place the eggs.

Put the flour into a third bowl.

Toss the cod fillets in the flour, then in the eggs, and then in the breadcrumb mixture.

Place them in the greased frying basket and AirFry for 9 minutes.

At the 5-minute mark, quickly turn the fillets.

Once done, remove to a plate and serve with cilantro-yogurt sauce.

Tandoori Crispy Salmon

Prep + Cook Time: 15 minutes

2 Serving

INGREDIENTS

2 salmon fillets

1 tsp ginger powder

1 garlic clove, minced

½ green bell pepper, sliced

1 tsp sweet paprika, minced

1 tsp honey

1 tsp garam masala

1 tbsp fresh cilantro, chopped

¼ cup yogurt

Juice and zest from

1 lime

DIRECTIONS

In a bowl, mix all the ingredients, except for salmon and yogurt.

Season to taste and stir in the yogurt.

Top the fillets with the mixture and let sit for 15 minutes.

Preheat air fryer to 400 F.

Place the fillets into the greased frying basket and Bake for 12-15 minutes until nice and crispy.

Serve on a bed of rice.

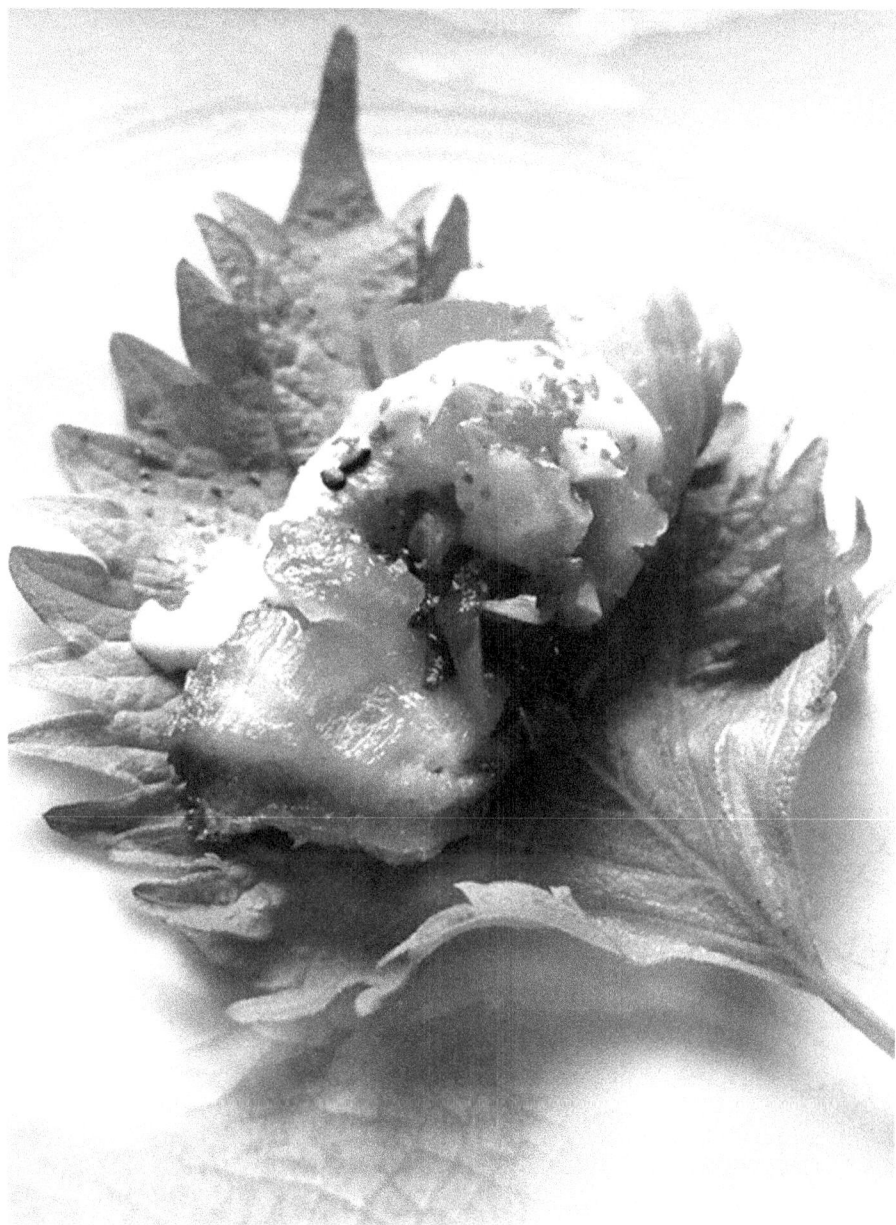

Smoked Salmon Taquitos

Prep + Cook Time: 15 minutes

4 Servings

INGREDIENTS

2 tbsp olive oil

1 lb smoked salmon, chopped

Salt to taste

1 tbsp taco seasoning

1 cup cheddar cheese, shredded

1 lime, juiced

½ cup fresh cilantro, chopped

8 corn tortillas

DIRECTIONS

Preheat air fryer to 390 F.

In a bowl, mix salmon, taco seasoning, lime juice, cheddar cheese, salt, and cilantro.

Divide the mixture between the tortillas.

Wrap the tortillas around the filling and place them in the greased air fryer basket.

Bake for 10 minutes, turning once halfway through.

Serve with hot salsa.

Lovely "Blackened" Catfish

Prep + Cook Time: 20 minutes

2 Servings

INGREDIENTS

2 catfish fillets

2 tsp blackening seasoning

Juice of 1 lime

2 tbsp butter, melted

1 garlic clove, minced

2 tbsp fresh cilantro, chopped

DIRECTIONS

Preheat air fryer to 360 F.

In a bowl, mix garlic, lime juice, cilantro, and butter.

Divide the sauce into two parts, rub 1 part of the sauce onto fish fillets and sprinkle with the seasoning.

Place the fillets in the greased frying basket and Bake for 15 minutes, flipping once. Serve with the remaining sauce.

Jamaican Catfish Fillets

Prep + Cook Time: 20 minutes

4 Servings

INGREDIENTS

4 catfish fillets

2 tbsp olive oil

1 tsp paprika

1 tsp garlic powder

1 tsp dried basil

1 tbsp ground Jamaican allspice

½ lemon, juiced

DIRECTIONS

Preheat air fryer to 390 F.

Spray the frying basket with cooking spray.

In a bowl, mix paprika, garlic powder, and Jamaican allspice seasoning.

Rub the catfish fillets with the spice mixture.

Transfer to the frying basket and drizzle the olive oil.

AirFry for 8 minutes, slide the basket out and turn the fillets.

Cook further for 5 minutes until crispy.

Sprinkle with lemon juice to serve.

Hot Sardine Cakes

Prep + Cook Time: 20 minutes

4 Servings

INGREDIENTS

2 4-oz tins sardines, chopped

2 eggs, beaten

½ cup breadcrumbs

⅓ cup green onions, finely chopped

2 tbsp fresh parsley, chopped

1 tbsp mayonnaise

1 tsp sweet chili sauce

½ tsp paprika

Salt and black pepper to taste

2 tbsp olive oil

DIRECTIONS

In a bowl, add sardines, eggs, breadcrumbs, green onions, parsley, mayonnaise, chili sauce, paprika, salt, and black pepper.

Mix well with hands.

Shape into 8 cakes and brush them lightly with olive oil.

AirFry in the fryer for 8 minutes at 390 F, shaking once halfway through cooking.

Serve warm.

Basil White Fish with Cheese

Prep + Cook Time: 15 minutes

4 Servings

INGREDIENTS

2 tbsp fresh basil, chopped

1 tsp garlic powder

2 tbsp Romano cheese, grated

Salt and black pepper to taste

4 white fish fillets

DIRECTIONS

Preheat air fryer to 350 F.

Season fillets with garlic, salt, and black pepper.

Place in the greased frying basket and AirFry them for 8-10 minutes, flipping once.

Serve topped with Romano cheese and basil.

Herbed Crab Croquettes

Prep + Cook Time: 25 minutes

4 Servings

INGREDIENTS

1 ½ lb lump crab meat

⅓ cup sour cream

⅓ cup mayonnaise

1 red pepper, finely chopped

⅓ cup red onion, chopped

½ celery stalk, chopped

1 tsp fresh tarragon, chopped

1 tsp fresh chives, chopped

1 tsp fresh parsley, chopped

1 tsp cayenne pepper

1 ½ cups breadcrumbs

2 tsp olive oil

1 cup flour

3 eggs, beaten

Salt to taste

Lemon wedges to serve

DIRECTIONS

Heat olive oil in a skillet over medium heat and sauté red pepper, onion, and celery for 5 minutes or until sweaty and translucent.

Turn off the heat.

Pour the breadcrumbs and salt on a plate.

In 2 separate bowls, add the flour and beaten eggs, respectively, set aside.

In a separate bowl, add crabmeat, mayo, sour cream, tarragon, chives, parsley, cayenne pepper, and vegetable sauteed mix.

Form bite-sized oval balls from the mixture and place them onto a plate. Preheat air fryer to 390 F.

Dip each crab meatball in the beaten eggs and press them in the breadcrumb mixture.

Place the croquettes in the greased fryer basket without overcrowding.

Cook for 10 minutes until golden brown, shaking once halfway through. Serve hot with lemon wedges.

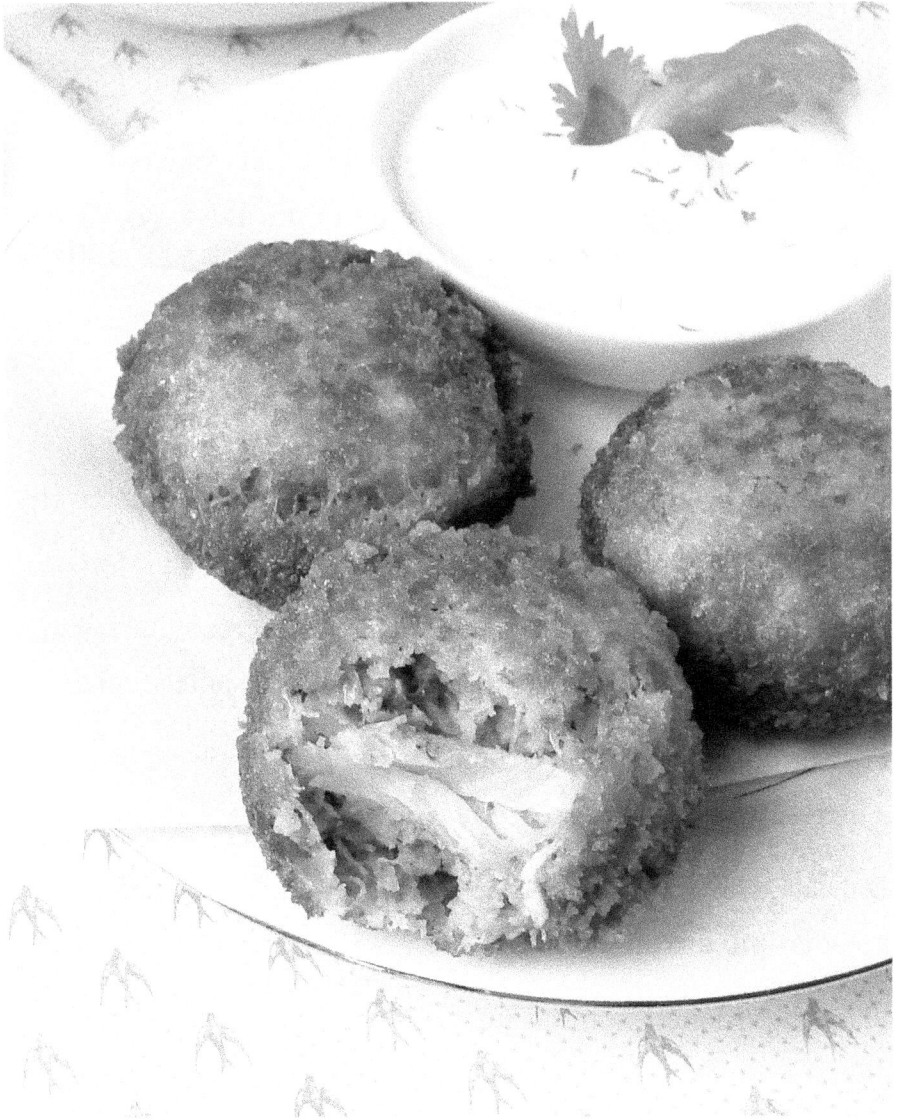

Chinese Garlic Prawns

Prep + Cook Time: 20 minutes + marinating time

4 Servings

INGREDIENTS

1 lb prawns, peeled and deveined

Juice of 1 lemon

1 tsp sugar

2 tbsp peanut oil

2 tbsp cornstarch

2 scallions, chopped

¼ tsp Chinese powder

1 red chili pepper, minced

Salt and black pepper to taste

4 garlic cloves, minced

DIRECTIONS

In a Ziploc bag, mix lemon juice, sugar, black pepper, 1 tbsp peanut oil, cornstarch, Chinese powder, and salt.

Add in prawns and massage gently to coat.

Let sit for 20 minutes.

Heat the remaining peanut oil in a pan over medium heat and sauté garlic, scallions, and red chili pepper for 5 minutes.

Preheat air fryer to 390 F.

Place the marinated prawns in a baking dish and cover with the sautéed vegetables.

AirFry for 10 minutes, shaking once halfway through, until nice and crispy.

Serve warm.

Cod Cornflakes Nuggets with Avocado Dip

Prep + Cook Time: 25 minutes

4 Servings

INGREDIENTS

1 ¼ lb cod fillets, cut into 4 chunks each

½ cup flour

2 eggs, beaten

1 cup cornflakes

1 tbsp olive oil

Salt and black pepper to taste

1 avocado, chopped

1 lime, juiced

DIRECTIONS

Mash the avocado with a fork in a small bowl.

Stir in lime juice and salt and set aside.

Place olive oil and cornflakes in a food processor and process until crumbed.

Season the fish with salt and pepper.

Preheat air fryer to 350 F.

Place flour, eggs and cornflakes in separate dishes.

Toss the fish with flour, dip in eggs, then coat well with cornflakes.

AirFry for 15 minutes until golden.

Serve with avocado dip.

Baked Trout en Papillote with Herbs

Prep + Cook Time: 20 minutes

2 Servings

INGREDIENTS

2 whole trout, scaled and cleaned

¼ bulb fennel, sliced

½ brown onion, sliced

1 tbsp fresh parsley, chopped

1 tbsp fresh dill, chopped

1 tbsp olive oil

1 lemon, sliced

Salt and black pepper to taste

DIRECTIONS

In a bowl, add the onion, parsley, dill, fennel, and garlic.

Mix and drizzle with olive oil.

Preheat air fryer to 350 F.

Open the cavity of the fish and fill with the fennel mixture.

Wrap the fish completely in parchment paper and then in foil.

Place the fish in the frying basket and Bake for 14 minutes.

Remove the paper and foil and top with lemon slices to serve

Ale-Battered Fish with Tartar Sauce

Prep + Cook Time: 20 minutes

4 Servings

INGREDIENTS

4 lemon wedges

2 eggs

1 cup ale beer

1 cup flour

Salt and black pepper to taste

4 white fish fillets

½ cup light mayonnaise

½ cup Greek yogurt

2 dill pickles, chopped

1 tbsp capers

1 tbsp fresh dill, roughly chopped

Lemon wedges to serve

DIRECTIONS

Preheat air fryer to 390 F.

Beat the eggs in a bowl along with ale beer, salt, and black pepper.

Pat dry the fish fillets with paper towels and dredge them in the flour.

Shake off the excess flour.

Dip in the egg mixture and then in the flour again.

Spray with cooking spray and add to the frying basket.

AirFry for 10 minutes, flipping once.

In a bowl, mix mayonnaise, yogurt, capers, salt, and dill pickles.

Serve the fish with the sauce and freshly cut lemon wedges.

Peppery & Lemony Haddock

Prep + Cook Time: 20 minutes

4 Servings

INGREDIENTS

4 haddock fillets

1 cup breadcrumbs

2 tbsp lemon juice

Salt and black pepper to taste

¼ cup potato flakes

2 eggs, beaten

¼ cup Parmesan cheese, grated

3 tbsp flour

DIRECTIONS

In a bowl, combine flour, salt, and pepper.

In another bowl, combine breadcrumbs, Parmesan cheese, and potato flakes.

Dip fillets in the flour first, then in the eggs, and coat them with the cheese crumbs.

Place in the frying basket and AirFry for 14-16 minutes at 370 F, flipping once.

Serve with lemon juice.

Oaty Fishcakes

Prep + Cook Time: 20 minutes

4 Servings

INGREDIENTS

4 potatoes, cooked and mashed

2 salmon fillets, cubed

1 haddock fillet, cubed

1 tsp Dijon mustard

½ cup oats

2 tbsp fresh dill, chopped

2 tbsp olive oil

Salt and black pepper to taste

DIRECTIONS

Preheat air fryer to 400 F.

Boil salmon and haddock cubes in a pot filled with salted water over medium heat for 5 minutes.

Drain, cool, and pat dry.

Flake or shred and add to a bowl.

Mix in mashed potatoes, mustard, oats, dill, salt, and pepper.

Shape into balls and flatten to make patties.

Brush with olive oil and arrange them on the bottom of the frying basket.

Bake for 10 minutes, flipping once halfway through.

Let cool before serving.

Fiery Prawns

Prep + Cook Time: 15 minutes

4 Servings

INGREDIENTS

8 prawns, cleaned

Salt and black pepper to taste

½ tsp ground cayenne pepper

½ tsp red chili flakes

½ tsp ground cumin

½ tsp garlic powder

DIRECTIONS

In a bowl, season the prawns with salt and black pepper.

Sprinkle with cayenne pepper, chili flakes, cumin, and garlic, and stir to coat.

Spray the frying basket with oil and lay the prawns in an even layer.

AirFry for 8 minutes at 340 F, turning once halfway through.

Serve with fresh sweet chili sauce.

Buttered Crab Legs

Prep + Cook Time: 15 minutes

4 Servings

INGREDIENTS

3 lb crab legs

2 tbsp butter, melted

1 tbsp fresh parsley

DIRECTIONS

Preheat air fryer to 380 F.

Place the crab legs in the greased air fryer basket and AirFry for 10 minutes, shaking once.

Pour the butter over crab legs, sprinkle with parsley, and serve.

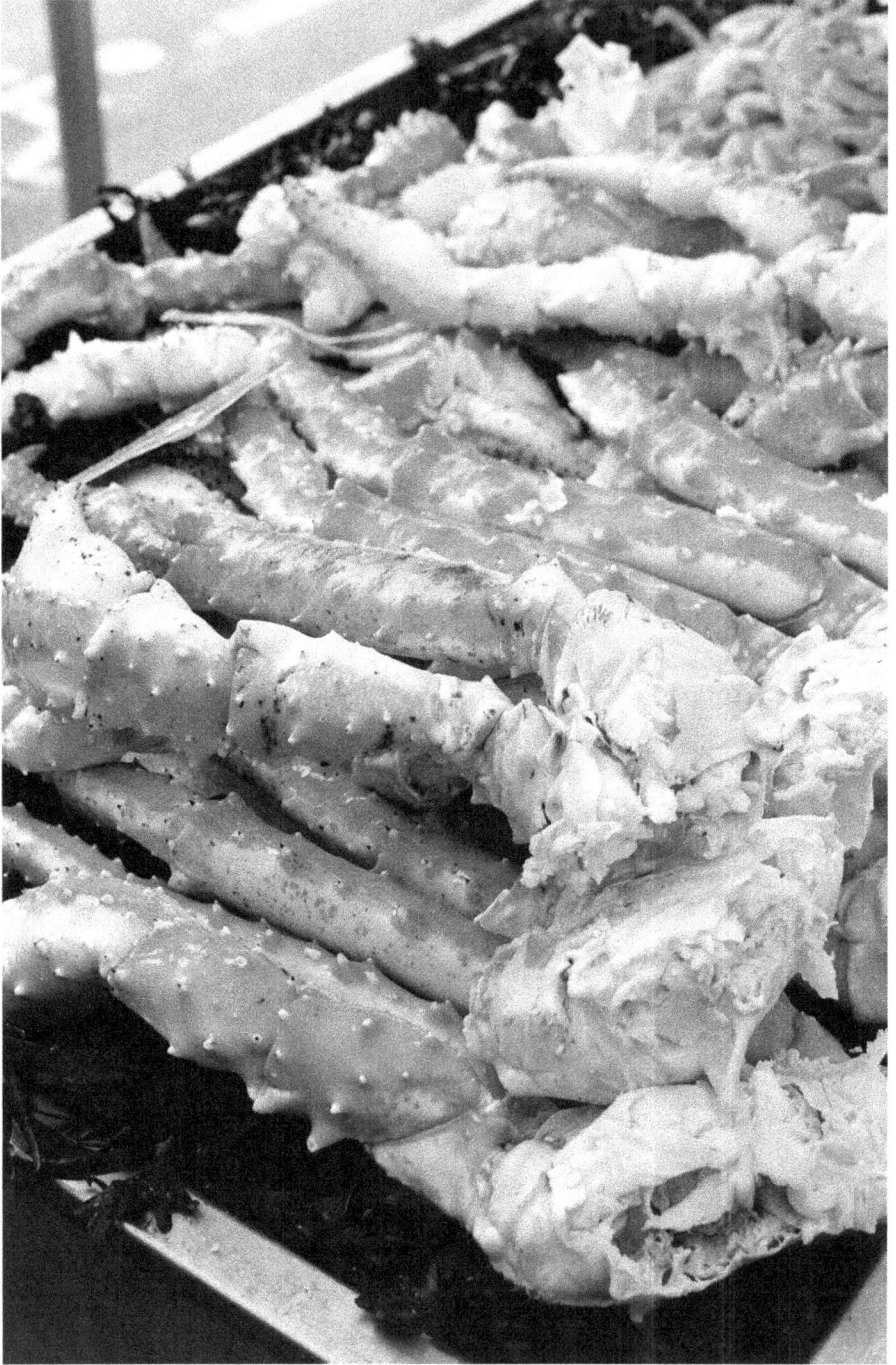

Air-Fried Seafood

Prep + Cook Time: 15 minutes

4 Servings

INGREDIENTS

1 lb fresh scallops, mussels, fish fillets, prawns, shrimp

2 eggs

 Salt and black pepper to taste

1 cup breadcrumbs mixed with the zest of 1 lemon

DIRECTIONS

Beat the eggs with salt and pepper in a bowl.

Dip in each piece of seafood and then coat with breadcrumbs.

Place in the greased air fryer basket and AirFry for 10-12 minutes at 400 F, turning once.

Cod Finger Pesto Sandwich

Prep + Cook Time: 20 minutes

4 Servings

INGREDIENTS

4 cod fillets

4 bread rolls

1 cup breadcrumbs

4 tbsp pesto sauce

4 lettuce leaves

Salt and black pepper to taste

DIRECTIONS

Preheat air fryer to 370 F.

Season the fillets with salt and black pepper and coat them with breadcrumbs.

Arrange them into the greased air fryer basket and Bake for 12-15 minutes, flipping once.

Cut the bread rolls in half.

Divide lettuce leaves between the bottom halves and place the fillets over.

Spread pesto sauce on top of the fillets and cover with the remaining halves to serve.

Hot Salmon Fillets with Broccoli

Prep + Cook Time: 25 minutes

2 Servings

INGREDIENTS

2 salmon fillets

2 tsp olive oil

Juice of 1 lime

1 tsp chili flakes

Salt and black pepper to taste

5 oz broccoli florets, steamed

1 tbsp soy sauce

DIRECTIONS

In a bowl, add half of the olive oil, lime juice, chili flakes, salt, and black pepper; rub the mixture onto fillets.

Lay the florets into your air fryer and drizzle with the remaining olive oil.

Arrange the fillets on top and Bake at 340 F for 14 minutes, flipping once.

Drizzle the florets with soy sauce and serve with fish.

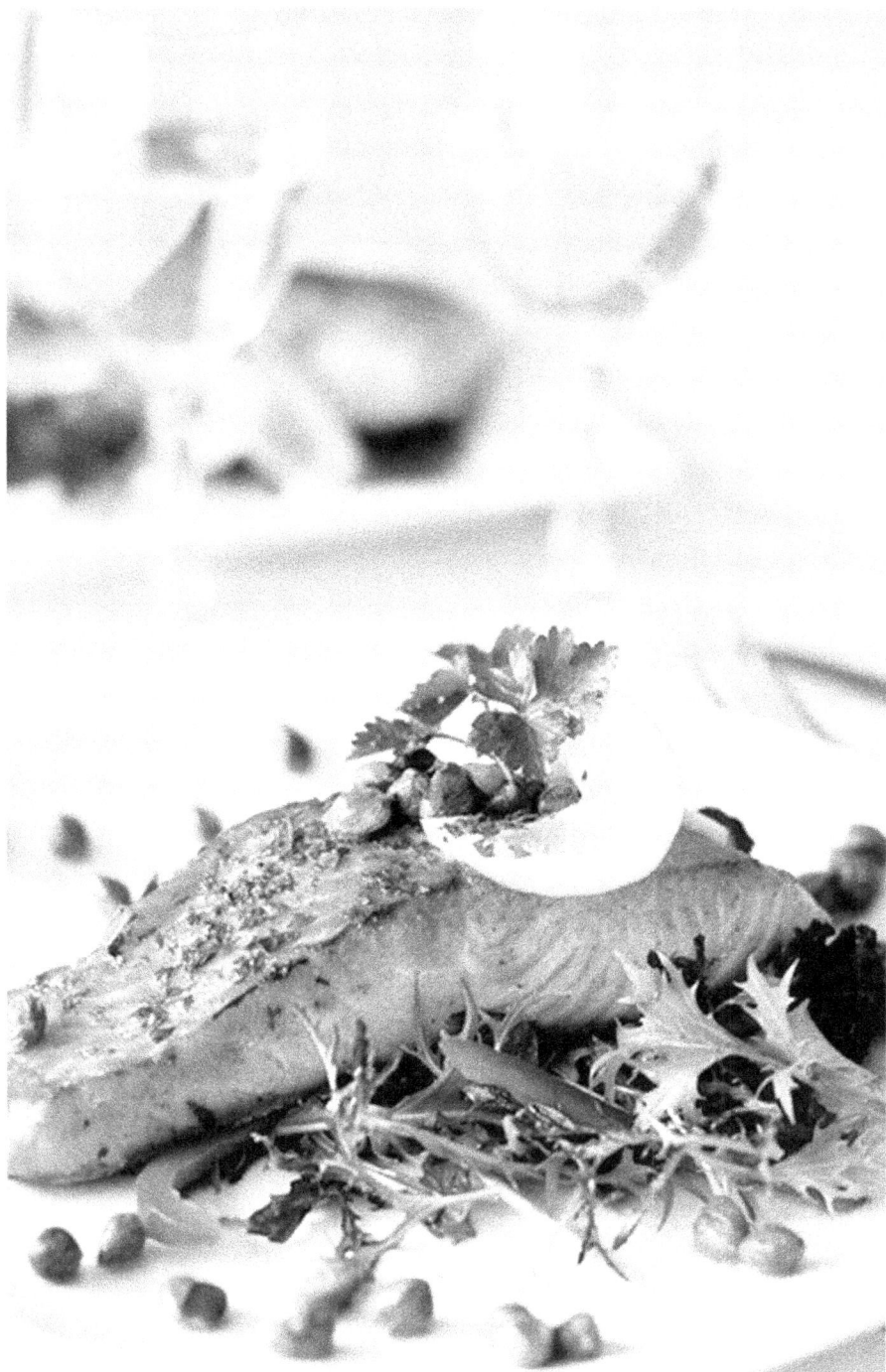

Crumbly Haddock Patties

Prep + Cook Time: 15 minutes + refrigerating time

2 Servings

INGREDIENTS

8 oz haddock, cooked and flaked

2 potatoes, cooked and mashed

2 tbsp green olives, pitted and chopped

1 tbsp fresh cilantro, chopped

1 tsp lemon zest

1 egg, beaten

DIRECTIONS

Mix haddock, zest, olives, cilantro, egg, and potatoes.

Shape into patties and chill for 60 minutes.

Preheat air fryer to 350 F.

Place the patties in the greased baking basket and AirFry for 12-14 minutes, flipping once halfway through cooking.

Serve with green salad.

Sesame Halibut Fillets

Prep + Cook Time: 20 minutes

4 Servings

INGREDIENTS

4 halibut fillets

4 biscuits, crumbled

3 tbsp flour

1 egg, beaten

Salt and black pepper to taste

¼ tsp dried rosemary

3 tbsp olive oil

2 tbsp sesame seeds

DIRECTIONS

Preheat air fryer to 390 F.

In a bowl, combine flour, black pepper, and salt.

In another bowl, combine sesame seeds, crumbled biscuits, olive oil, and rosemary.

Dip the fish fillets into the flour mixture first, then into the beaten egg.

Finally, coat them with the sesame mixture.

Arrange on the greased frying basket and AirFry for 8 minutes.

Flip the fillets and cook for 4-5 more minutes.

Serve immediately.

Delicious Coconut Shrimp

Prep + Cook Time: 30 minutes

2 Servings

INGREDIENTS

8 large shrimp, peeled and deveined

½ cup breadcrumbs

8 oz coconut milk

½ cup coconut, shredded

Salt to taste

½ cup orange jam

1 tsp mustard

1 tbsp honey

½ tsp cayenne pepper

¼ tsp hot sauce

DIRECTIONS

Combine breadcrumbs, cayenne pepper, shredded coconut, and salt in a bowl.

Dip the shrimp in the coconut milk, and then in the coconut crumbs.

Arrange on a lined sheet and Bake in the air fryer for 12 minutes at 350 F.

Whisk jam, honey, hot sauce, and mustard in a bowl.

Serve with the shrimp.

Asian Shrimp Medley

Prep + Cook Time: 20 minutes + marinating time

4 Servings

INGREDIENTS

1 lb shrimp, peeled and deveined

2 whole onions, chopped

3 tbsp butter

1 tbsp sugar

2 tbsp soy sauce

2 cloves garlic, chopped

2 tsp lime juice

1 tsp ginger paste

DIRECTIONS

Melt butter in a frying pan over medium heat and stir-fry the onions for 3 minutes until translucent.

Mix in the lime juice, soy sauce, ginger paste, garlic, and sugar and stir for 1-2 minutes.

Let cool and then pour the mixture over the shrimp.

Cover and let marinate for 30 minutes in the fridge.

Preheat air fryer to 380 F.

Transfer the shrimp with marinade to a baking dish and AirFry in the fryer for 12 minutes, shaking once halfway through.

Serve warm.

Breaded Scallops

Prep + Cook Time: 10 minutes

4 Servings

INGREDIENTS

1 lb fresh scallops

3 tbsp flour

Salt and black pepper to taste

1 egg, lightly beaten

1 cup breadcrumbs

2 tbsp olive oil

½ tsp fresh parsley, chopped

DIRECTIONS

Coat the scallops with flour.

Dip into the egg, then into the breadcrumbs.

Brush with olive oil and place into the frying basket.

AirFry for 6-8 minutes at 360 F, shaking once.

Serve topped with parsley. Enjoy!

Kimchi-Spiced Salmon

Prep + Cook Time: 15 minutes

4 Servings

INGREDIENTS

2 tbsp soy sauce

2 tbsp sesame oil

2 tbsp mirin

1 tbsp ginger puree

1 tsp kimchi spice

1 tsp sriracha sauce

2 lb salmon fillets

1 lime, cut into wedges

DIRECTIONS

Preheat air fryer to 350 F.

Grease the air fryer basket with cooking spray.

In a bowl, mix together soy sauce, mirin, ginger puree, kimchi spice, and sriracha sauce.

Add the salmon fillets and toss to coat.

Place in the air fryer basket and drizzle with sesame oil.

AirFry for 10 minutes, flipping once halfway through.

Garnish with lime wedges and serve

Mediterranean Salmon

Prep + Cook Time: 15 minutes

2 Servings

INGREDIENTS

2 salmon fillets

Salt and black pepper to taste

1 lemon, cut into wedges

8 asparagus spears, trimmed

DIRECTIONS

Rinse and pat dry the fillets with a paper towel.

Coat the fish generously on both sides with cooking spray.

Season fish and asparagus with salt and pepper.

Arrange fish in the frying basket and lay the asparagus around the fish.

AirFry for 10-12 minutes at 350 F, flipping once.

Serve with lemon wedges.

Air Fried Tuna Sandwich

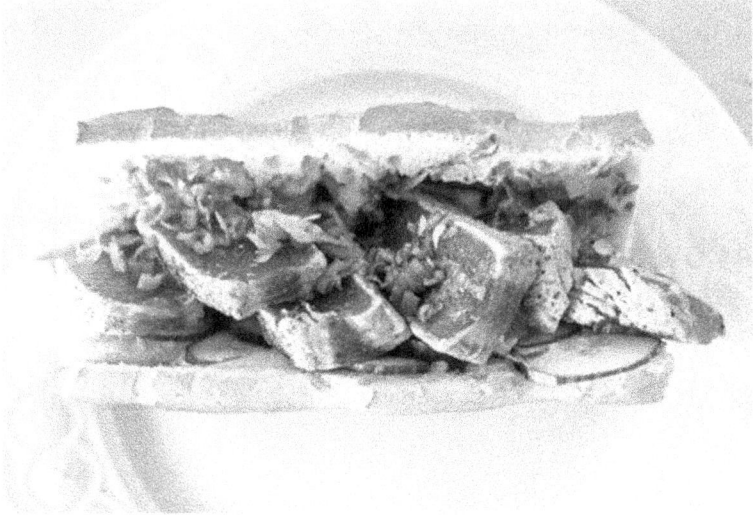

Prep + Cook Time: 10 minutes

2 Servings

INGREDIENTS

4 white bread slices

1 5-oz can tuna, drained

½ onion, finely chopped

2 tbsp mayonnaise

1 cup mozzarella cheese, shredded

1 tbsp olive oil

DIRECTIONS

In a small bowl, mix tuna, onion, and mayonnaise.

Spoon the mixture over two bread slices, top with mozzarella cheese, and cover with the remaining bread slices.

Brush with olive oil and arrange the sandwiches in the air fryer basket.

Bake at 360 F for 6-8 minutes, turning once halfway through.

Serve and enjoy!

Greek-Style Fried Mussels

Prep + Cook Time: 30 minutes

4 Servings

INGREDIENTS

4 lb mussels

4 tbsp olive oil

1 cup white wine

Salt and black pepper to taste

1 tsp Greek seasoning

2 tbsp white wine vinegar

5 garlic cloves

4 bread slices

½ cup mixed nuts

DIRECTIONS

Preheat air fryer to 350 F.

Add olive oil, garlic, Greek seasoning, vinegar, salt, mixed nuts, black pepper, and bread slices to a food processor and process until you obtain a creamy texture.

In a skillet over medium heat, add wine and mussels.

Bring to a boil, then lower the heat and simmer until the mussels have opened up.

Then, drain and remove from the shells.

Add them to the previously prepared mixture and toss to coat.

Place in a greased baking dish and Bake in the air fryer for 10 minutes, shaking once.

Serve warm.

Greek-Style Salmon with Dill Sauce

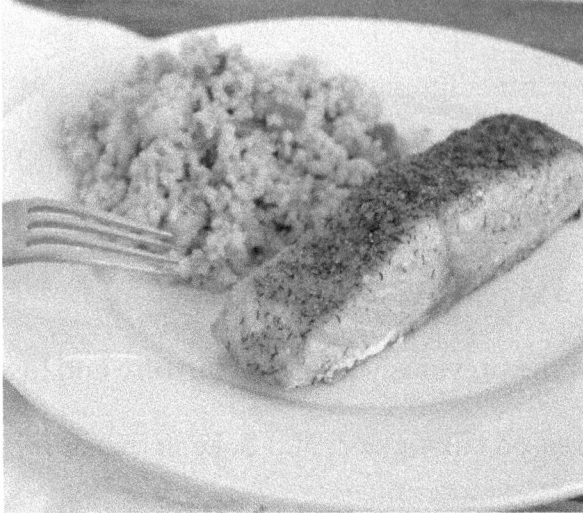

Prep + Cook Time: 20 minutes

4 Servings

INGREDIENTS

1 lb salmon fillets

Salt and black pepper to taste

2 tsp olive oil

2 tbsp fresh dill, chopped

1 cup sour cream

1 cup Greek yogurt

DIRECTIONS

In a bowl, mix sour cream, yogurt, dill, and salt; set aside. Preheat air fryer to 340 F.

Drizzle olive oil over the salmon and rub with salt and black pepper.

Arrange the fish in the frying basket and Bake for 10 minutes, flipping once.

Top with the yogurt sauce.

Simple Creole Trout

Prep + Cook Time: 15 minutes

4 Servings

INGREDIENTS

4 skin-on trout fillets

2 tsp creole seasoning

2 tbsp fresh dill, chopped

1 lemon, sliced

DIRECTIONS

Preheat air fryer to 350 F.

Season the trout with creole seasoning on both sides and spray with cooking spray.

Place in the frying basket and Bake for 10-12 minutes, flipping once.

Serve sprinkled with dill and garnished with lemon slices. Enjoy!

Colorful Salmon and Fennel Salad

Prep + Cook Time: 20 minutes

3 Servings

INGREDIENTS

1 pound salmon

1 fennel, quartered

1 teaspoon olive oil

Sea salt and ground black pepper, to taste

1/2 teaspoon paprika

1 tablespoon balsamic vinegar

1 tablespoon lime juice

1 tablespoon extra-virgin olive oil

1 tomato, sliced

1 cucumber, sliced

1 tablespoon sesame seeds, lightly toasted

DIRECTIONS

Toss the salmon and fennel with 1 teaspoon of olive oil, salt, black pepper and paprika.

Cook in the preheated Air Fryer at 380 degrees F for 12 minutes; shaking the basket once or twice.

Cut the salmon into bite-sized strips and transfer them to a nice salad bowl.

Add in the fennel, balsamic vinegar, lime juice, 1 tablespoon of extra-virgin olive oil, tomato and cucumber.

Toss to combine well and serve garnished with lightly toasted sesame seeds.

Enjoy!

Fish Sticks with Vidalia Onions

Prep + Cook Time: 12 minutes

2 Servings

INGREDIENTS

1/2 pound fish sticks, frozen

1/2 pound Vidalia onions, halved

1 teaspoon sesame oil

Sea salt and ground black pepper, to taste

1/2 teaspoon red pepper flakes

4 tablespoons mayonnaise

4 tablespoons Greek-style yogurt

1/4 teaspoon mustard seeds

1 teaspoon chipotle chili in adobo, minced

DIRECTIONS

Drizzle the fish sticks and Vidalia onions with sesame oil.

Toss them with salt, black pepper and red pepper flakes.

Transfer them to the Air Fryer cooking basket.

Cook the fish sticks and onions at 400 degreed F for 5 minutes.

Shake the basket and cook an additional 5 minutes or until cooked through.

Meanwhile, mix the mayonnaise, Greek- style yogurt, mustard seeds and chipotle chili.

Serve the warm fish sticks garnished with Vidalia onions and the sauce on the side.

Serve and enjoy!

Fish Cakes with Bell Pepper

Prep + Cook Time: 15 minutes 3 Servings INGREDIENTS

1 pound haddock

1 egg

2 tablespoons milk

1 bell pepper, deveined and finely chopped

2 stalks fresh scallions, minced

1/2 teaspoon fresh garlic, minced

Sea salt and ground black pepper, to taste

1/2 teaspoon cumin seeds

1/4 teaspoon celery seeds

1/2 cup breadcrumbs

1 teaspoon olive oil

DIRECTIONS

Thoroughly combine all ingredients, except for the breadcrumbs and olive oil, until everything is blended well.

Then, roll the mixture into 3 patties and coat them with breadcrumbs, pressing to adhere.

Drizzle olive oil over the patties and transfer them to the Air Fryer cooking basket.

Cook the fish cakes at 400 degrees F for 5 minutes; turn them over and continue to cook an additional 5 minutes until cooked through.

Serve and enjoy!

Cajun Fish Cakes with Cheese

Prep + Cook Time: 30 minutes

4 Servings

INGREDIENTS

2 catfish fillets

1 cup all-purpose flour

3 ounces butter

1 teaspoon baking powder

1 teaspoon baking soda

1/2 cup buttermilk

1 teaspoon Cajun seasoning

1 cup Swiss cheese, shredded

DIRECTIONS

Bring a pot of salted water to a boil.

Boil the fish fillets for 5 minutes or until it is opaque.

Flake the fish into small pieces.

Mix the remaining ingredients in a bowl; add the fish and mix until well combined.

Shape the fish mixture into 12 patties.

Cook in the preheated Air Fryer at 380 degrees F for 15 minutes.

Work in batches.

Enjoy!

Monkfish with Sautéed Vegetables and Olives

Prep + Cook Time: 20 minutes

2 Servings

INGREDIENTS

2 teaspoons olive oil

2 carrots, sliced

2 bell peppers, sliced

1 teaspoon dried thyme

1/2 teaspoon dried marjoram

1/2 teaspoon dried rosemary

2 monkfish fillets

1 tablespoon soy sauce

2 tablespoons lime juice

Coarse Salt and ground black pepper, to taste

1 teaspoon cayenne pepper

1/2 cup Kalamata olives, pitted and sliced

DIRECTIONS

In a nonstick skillet, heat the olive oil for 1 minute.

Once hot, sauté the carrots and peppers until tender, about 4 minutes.

Sprinkle with thyme, marjoram, and rosemary and set aside.

Toss the fish fillets with the soy sauce, lime juice, salt, black pepper, and cayenne pepper.

Place the fish fillets in a lightly greased cooking basket and bake at 390 degrees F for 8 minutes.

Turn them over, add the olives, and cook an additional 4 minutes.

Serve with the sautéed vegetables on the side.

Enjoy!

Crispy Mustardy Fish Fingers

Prep + Cook Time: 20 minutes

4 Servings

INGREDIENTS

1 ½ pounds tilapia pieces fingers

1/2 cup all-purpose flour

2 eggs

1 tablespoon yellow mustard

1 cup cornmeal

1 teaspoon garlic powder

1 teaspoon onion powder

Sea salt and ground black pepper, to taste

1/2 teaspoon celery powder

2 tablespoons peanut oil

DIRECTIONS

Pat dry the fish fingers with a kitchen towel.

To make a breading station, place the all-purpose flour in a shallow dish.

In a separate dish, whisk the eggs with mustard.

In a third bowl, mix the remaining ingredients.

Dredge the fish fingers in the flour, shaking the excess into the bowl; dip in the egg mixture and turn to coat evenly; then, dredge in the cornmeal mixture, turning a couple of times to coat evenly.

Cook in the preheated Air Fryer at 390 degrees F for 5 minutes; turn them over and cook another 5 minutes.

Enjoy!

Roasted Mediterranean Snapper Fillets

Prep + Cook Time: 20 minutes + Marinating Time

3 Servings

INGREDIENTS

Marinade:

1 tablespoon black olives, chopped

1/4 cup dry white wine

2 tablespoons fresh lemon juice

1/2 teaspoon dried oregano

1/2 teaspoon dried basil

1 tablespoon parsley leaves, chopped

1 tomato, pureed

Roasted Snapper:

1 pound snapper fillets

1/2 cup cassava flour

Salt and white pepper, to taste

DIRECTIONS

Add all ingredients for the marinade to a large ceramic bowl.

Add the snapper fillets and let them marinate for 1 hour in your refrigerator.

Place the cassava flour on a tray; now, coat the snapper fillets with the cassava flour.

Season with salt and pepper.

Cook the snapper fillets in the preheated Air Fryer at 395 degrees F for 10 minutes, basting with the marinade and flipping them halfway through the cooking time.

Serve and enjoy!

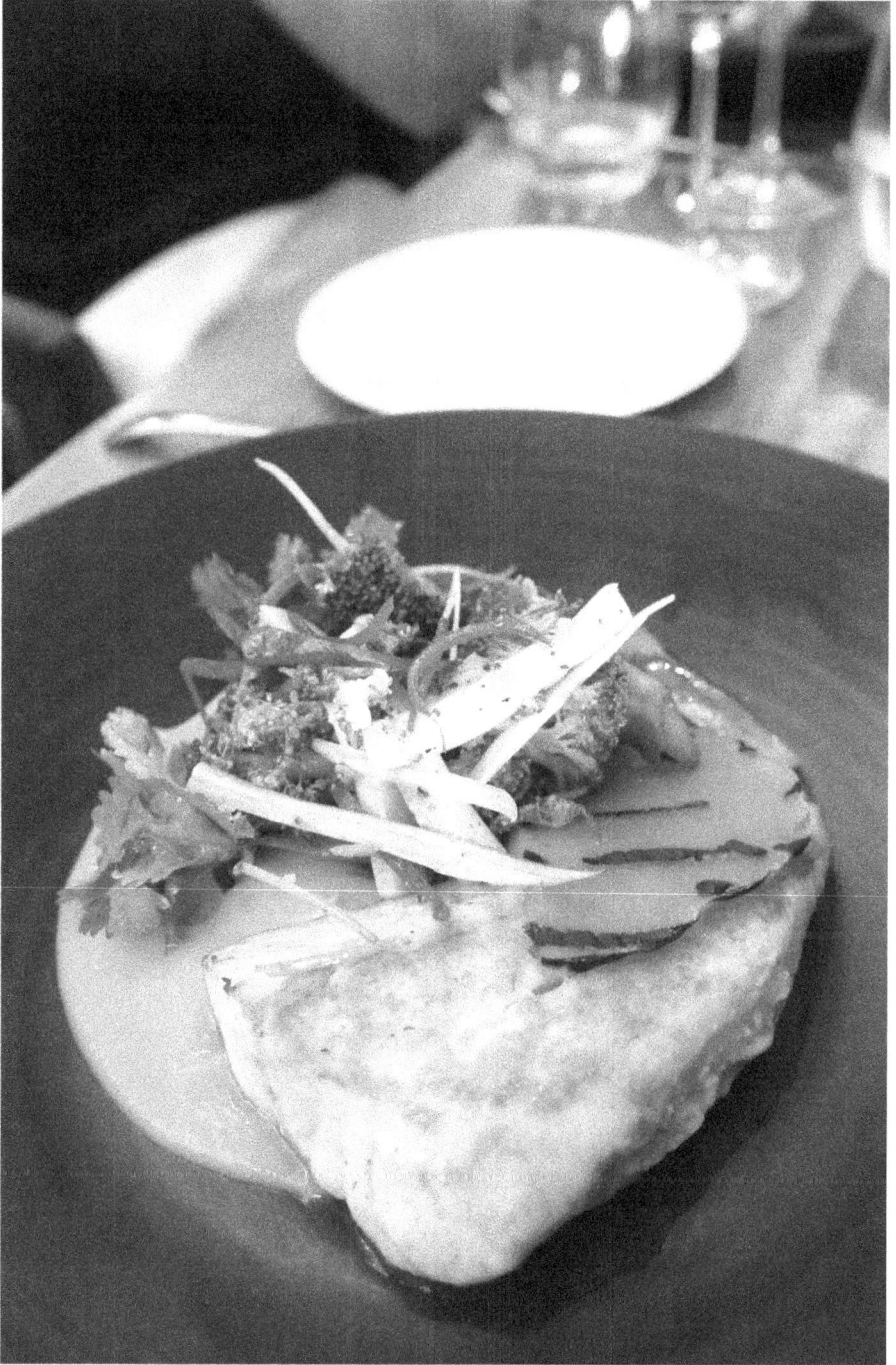

www.ingramcontent.com/pod-product-compliance
Lightning Source LLC
Chambersburg PA
CBHW071110030426
42336CB00013BA/2028